CW00505042

VETEI
ADVICE ON

SKIN

DISORDERS

IN DOGS

Tim Nuttall BSc, BVSc, PhD,
Cert VD, CBiol, MIBiol, MRCVS

ABOUT THE AUTHOR

Tim Nuttall graduated in Zoology and Veterinary Science from the University of Bristol in 1992. After three years in practice, he joined the Royal School of Veterinary Studies in Edinburgh where he passed the Royal College of Veterinary Surgeons' Certificate in Veterinary Dermatology in 1996. While at Edinburgh, he developed a particular interest in ear disease and yeast infections, and completed a PhD studying atopic dermatitis. Tim joined the University of Liverpool as Lecturer in Veterinary Dermatology in October 2001, where he sees clinical cases and continues research into the causes and treatment of allergic diseases. Tim has presented at national and international meetings, has written for a number of journals on skin diseaes, and is a founder member of the Pet Allergy Association (www.petallergy.org.uk).

ACKNOWLEDGEMENTS

Many thanks to Hill's Pet Nutrition for the use of its *Atlas of Veterinary Clinical Anatomy* for the line-drawing on page 44. Thanks also to: Viv Rainsbury: illustrations (page 6); Tim Nuttall: photographs (pages 3, 11, 13, 21, 24, 26, 27, 31, 36); Merial Animal Health: photograph (page 17); *Journal of Small Animal Practice*: photograph (page 43); *UK Vet*, Blackwell Scientific Publications, for the photographs on page 46 .

Published by Ringpress Books,
a division of Interpet Publishing,
Vincent Lane, Dorking, Surrey, RH4 3YX, UK.
Tel: 01306 873822   Fax: 01306 876712
email: sales@interpet.co.uk

First published 2004
© 2004 Ringpress Books. All rights reserved.

ISBN 1 86054 232 8

Printed and bound in Singapore by Kyodo Printing

10 9 8 7 6 5 4 3 2 1

CONTENTS

Introduction

S kin diseases are very common – possibly the most common group of diseases to affect dogs. Most diseases are not fatal, but they are often serious and debilitating. Furthermore, many become long-standing problems, requiring specialist treatment.

The skin can respond to problems in only a limited number of ways, which is why many skin diseases look alike. Skin diseases are often grouped according to the problems they cause. These groups include:

- Itching (also called pruritus)
- Hair loss (also called alopecia)
- Scaling
- Erosions and ulcers
- Changes in coloration
- Lumps and bumps.

Skin diseases can present with more than one problem, but there is invariably one overriding clinical sign – for example, an itchy dog might also have some secondary hair loss. The most prominent problem (in this case, itching) should be investigated first.

VETERINARY CARE

Dogs with any of the problems mentioned above should see their veterinary surgeon. Unfortunately, relatively few skin diseases can be diagnosed on the first visit, and many will require several visits, diagnostic tests or trial therapy. Most veterinary surgeons can deal with the usual skin complaints, but there may be situations where referral to a veterinary dermatologist (veterinary skin specialist) is needed. This is similar to a GP referring a patient to a consultant to make use of their greater knowledge and experience, facilities and equipment.

VETERINARY DERMATOLOGISTS

These are veterinary surgeons with a special interest and further qualifications in dermatology (the care of skin diseases). The Royal College of Veterinary Surgeons in the United Kingdom has a two-stage training programme leading to the Certificate and Diploma in Veterinary Dermatology (CertVD and DVD respectively). Veterinary dermatologists may also have Diplomas of the European and American Colleges of Veterinary Dermatology (DECVD and DACVD respectively). Veterinary dermatologists work in both private practice and university veterinary schools. Referrals can be made only through your own veterinary surgeon, who will either suggest a referral or arrange one at your request.

POSITIVE OUTLOOK

It is important to remember that, while some skin diseases can be very unpleasant, many can be well managed with the right care. If you suspect your dog has a skin disorder, it is important that you seek veterinary attention immediately. The sooner the problem is diagnosed, the greater the chances of curing or managing it and helping your dog to lead a normal life.

1 Skin structure and function

The skin is the largest organ in the body, shielding it from the potentially hostile world outside. It retains water and essential salts, excludes harmful microbes and parasites, and protects against injury.

LAYERS OF THE SKIN

- **Subcutis:** A fatty layer that insulates and shapes the body. Subcutaneous fat is an important vitamin reservoir. Vitamin D is partly synthesised in skin exposed to sunlight.
- **Dermis:** A network of fibres in a gel-like matrix that makes the skin tough, flexible and elastic. It contains all the blood vessels and nerves to the skin, as well as cells important for inflammation, repair, coat and skin colour, glands and secretions, and hair follicles.
- **Epidermis:** Forms a tough, waterproof barrier. Cells at the base of the epidermis continually divide, migrate outwards, and are shed from the surface.

CROSS-SECTION OF SKIN

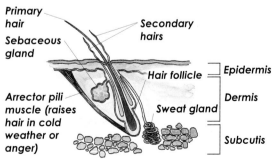

Primary hair

Secondary hairs

Sebaceous gland

Hair follicle — Epidermis

Arrector pili muscle (raises hair in cold weather or anger)

Sweat gland

Dermis

Subcutis

Many diseases trigger rapid cell division and skin thickening.

COAT TYPES AND HAIR FOLLICLES

Hair follicles are found in the dermis (everywhere except the nose and footpads). Each hair follicle goes through three phases – growing, transition and resting.

New, growing hairs eventually push out the old, resting hairs. Most dogs moult and grow a new coat each season, although there are exceptions (e.g. Poodles and Arctic breeds). However, dogs exposed to artificial light indoors tend to shed hairs all year round. All dog breeds essentially have one of three types of coat:

- Double: Coarse primary (or guard) hairs and a dense undercoat of fine, secondary hairs (e.g. German Shepherd Dog).
- Short: Uniform hairs comprising primary (Rottweiler) or secondary hairs (smooth-haired Dachshund).
- Long: These are made up of uniformly long, fine (Cocker Spaniel) or woolly (Poodle) secondary hairs.

Hair follicles are normally at an angle within the skin, allowing the coat to lie naturally from head to tail. Small muscles attached to the base of each follicle can pull them upright, raising the hairs. This increases insulation in cold weather. 'Raised hackles' are also an important social signal.

Whiskers are specialised hairs, longer and thicker than ordinary hairs. Found on the muzzle and the face, they are exquisitely sensitive to touch. Small, whisker-like hairs, also sensitive to touch, are scattered throughout the coat.

COAT AND SKIN COLOUR

Pigments (melanins) determine colour. There are two types of melanins in dogs – black/brown and yellow-red. The final colour depends on the relative abundance and distribution of these melanins. Other coats are self-coloured (single colour) or piebald (distribution of different colours). Genetic control of colour is complex, and many colours do not breed true.

SEBUM AND SWEAT

Sebum is secreted by sebaceous glands. It helps to bind epidermal cells, provides them with nutrients, contains antibodies, prevents the skin and hairs from drying out, and gives the coat its sheen. While dogs have sweat glands, these are not used to regulate temperature as in humans. Instead, sweat forms part of sebum and eliminates waste products.

SPECIALISED SKIN

The skin of the nose and the footpads is hairless, very thick, and tightly attached to underlying tissues. This makes these sites very tough and resilient. Nails are also classified as specialised skin. The skin over the last toe bone produces a very thick, hard form of epidermis, stronger (but less flexible) than the epidermis elsewhere.

SUMMARY – FUNCTIONS OF THE SKIN
- Tough outer barrier providing shape and form
- Immune system protects against infection
- Protection against UV radiation
- Temperature regulation
- Sensations of touch, pressure, itch, pain and heat
- Eliminates waste products
- Stores fat and vitamins
- Produces vitamin D.

2 Routine skin care

For most healthy dogs, routine skin care is quite straightforward. Basic grooming is essential – it removes dead hairs and cells, matted hairs, and debris, and stimulates blood flow to the skin, promoting normal skin and hair growth. It also reinforces the bond between dog and owner.

Long-haired dogs need extra attention, but all dogs should be groomed each day. It is easier to spend 5-10 minutes grooming each day, than to attack a matted coat for an hour every fortnight!

Grooming parlours are generally very good, but they are not an alternative to grooming at home. Most dogs are relatively easy to groom, but if you have never tried before, consult your vet, breeder or a good-quality grooming guide.

HAIRLESS DOGS

Some breeds are born hairless, while others lose hair as they age. The underlying skin is often thickened, oily or scaly and in need of care. Vigorous massaging loosens scale, removes excess skin and promotes healthy blood flow. Degreasing shampoos counter excessive oiliness, but depending on your dog's skin type, you may need to use a moisturiser afterwards.

Hairless dogs also need coats in cold weather and protection from strong sunlight. Exposure to strong sunlight can cause sunburn and skin cancers in hairless dogs or dogs with sparse coats, light-coloured skin or scars. Some steps can be taken to protect them:

• Keep dogs indoors when the sun is strongest.

- Hats, T-shirts, shorts and goggles can be customised for dogs. Commercial body suits are also available.
- Black marker pen can protect small areas of skin. Tattooing isn't helpful, as the dye goes under the skin.
- Sun blocks are useful, but dogs tend to lick them off. High-SPF (sun protection factor) sports blocks that are waterproof and sweat-resistant are best, but they should be applied frequently.

BATHING

Some skin conditions benefit from regular bathing. Mild, moisturising shampoos suitable for dogs are available from veterinary surgeries. These can also be used to treat dry skins or to counter over-drying caused by some medicated shampoos.

Medicated shampoos are useful for treating infections, parasites, dry or greasy scaling, and inflamed or itchy skins. Remember that it is very important to follow the manufacturer's instructions.

Always use veterinary shampoos designed for them, however, as human shampoos are too harsh for dogs. If you have never bathed a dog before, discuss it with your vet. Some veterinary practices and grooming parlours offer regular bathing clinics.

Whirlpool baths are excellent, but good results can be obtained using shower attachments in ordinary baths. Do not use garden hoses – these can be distressing for all concerned.

In most cases, dogs should be bathed two to three times a week once treatment commences. Once the skin problem is under control, the regularity of bathing or the type of product used can be changed in consultation with your vet. Stop treatment and see your vet if your dog develops any new irritation.

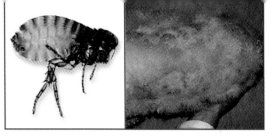

Despite its size, the tiny flea (left) can be responsible for a range of skin disorders, one of the most common being flea-allergic dermatitis (right).

FLEAS

Flea control is a subject all dog owners must understand, and it must form part of your regular grooming routine. For dogs with skin problems, flea control is even more important, as reaction to flea bites can worsen an existing skin condition. Fleas can cause itching, inflammation and crusting, especially over the back, hind legs and flanks. Secondary infections and intense self-trauma are common. Fleas also pass on the tapeworm *Dipylidium caninum*. Tests can identify flea allergies (see Chapter Three).

LIFE CYCLE

The flea life cycle takes about three weeks indoors, although eggs and pupae can lie dormant for some months if conditions aren't right.

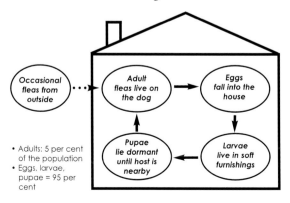

Occasional fleas from outside

Adult fleas live on the dog

Eggs fall into the house

Pupae lie dormant until host is nearby

Larvae live in soft furnishings

- Adults: 5 per cent of the population
- Eggs, larvae, pupae = 95 per cent

FLEA CONTROL

Modern prescription insecticides are highly specific to fleas and much less toxic than they used to be. Most are available as spot-on treatments or drops, normally administered once every one to three months. Insect growth regulators block flea growth and development, preventing viable eggs being laid. They are now available as tablets and drops, and are very safe.

Non-prescription products (e.g. powders and shampoos) are less effective. Flea collars are best avoided, as they can cause reactions. Your vet will advise you on the most suitable products for your dog.

Remember to follow instructions carefully. Also remember to treat all your pets (particularly cats), and ensure that any visiting animals have also been treated.

Flea-allergic animals are the most difficult cases to manage, as even a very small number of flea bites can provoke a reaction. Ideally, you should use both highly effective spot-on treatments and environmental treatments in combination. Your vet will advise you.

As well as treating your dog, you will need to treat your home. Sprays containing both an insecticide to kill adults and an insect growth regulator to break the life cycle will protect your home for 6-12 months. Everywhere must be treated, which might even include the car!

- Vacuum before and after treatment. Spray vacuum bags, or put a flea collar inside, to kill fleas picked up.
- Thoroughly spray all carpets and soft furnishings. Pay particular attention to your pet's favourite haunts. Bedding can be washed at high temperatures.
- Air rooms after spraying and follow instructions and safety precautions carefully.
- Treating a house is a considerable undertaking. Local authorities may treat heavily infested homes.

3 Diagnosing skin problems

Many skin diseases cannot be diagnosed on a single visit, and tests are often necessary to confirm the diagnosis. Most, however, are quick, easy procedures that cause little discomfort.

COAT BRUSHINGS
Run a fine-toothed comb through the coat and examine the collected material with a hand lens on white paper.
- Fleas are thin, dark brown insects that jump! Unlike soil, flea dirt is dark purple, shiny, and leaves a reddish stain on damp, white paper.
- Lice are large, slow-moving, whitish insects that cling to the hairs. Look for their eggs ('nits') stuck to hairs.
- *Cheyletiella* mites can be seen as tiny white specks moving on dark paper – hence the term 'walking dandruff'. Their eggs are also stuck to hairs, but are much smaller than louse eggs.

FUNGAL SPORES
Fungal spores are routinely collected by running a toothbrush through the coat and sending the head of the brush away for culture (see page 15).

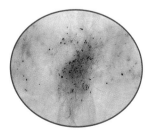

Run a fine-toothed comb through your dog's coat and collect the results on some tissue. Flea faeces are semi-digested blood, and they will leave a red-brown stain on damp tissue.

SKIN SCRAPES

Skin scrapes are usually carried out when looking for mites. Superficial skin layers are scraped on to a glass slide using a scalpel blade. The collected material is then examined using a microscope. Skin scrapes leave a graze that quickly heals. Most dogs tolerate skin scrapes very well, but excitable dogs may need some sedation.

HAIR PLUCKS

The hairs are firmly grasped by forceps, pulled out, and looked at under a microscope for fungal infections, parasites, the stage of the hair cycle, and hair shaft defects. Plucking causes only momentary discomfort.

CYTOLOGY

Cytology is the science of looking at cells. Cells from the skin surface are collected using glass slides or swabs, whereas a needle and syringe are used to collect cells from deeper lesions. Cytology is an inexpensive, quick technique that dogs tolerate very well. It is very good at detecting infections, inflammation, abnormal cells and cancers, but does not always yield accurate or complete results, as only a few cells are ever looked at. Ear swabs are particularly informative and can identify ear mites, bacterial or yeast infections. Cytology samples can either be examined in the veterinary practice or sent away for analysis.

SKIN BIOPSY

Skin biopsies tell us how cells interact with each other and the skin. They are more accurate than cytology, but also more invasive. Skin biopsies are routine when diagnosing inflammatory diseases, tumours and hair loss.

Dogs are usually sedated to keep them still, and a

local anaesthetic is injected under the skin. A small cylinder of skin (4-8 mm diameter) is removed with a punch and the skin edges sutured together. Several biopsies from different sites are often taken if there is widespread disease. A general anaesthetic is usually given for biopsies from very sensitive sites, such as the feet or face.

BLOOD SAMPLES

Blood samples are usually taken from the jugular vein in the neck. Samples can be analysed by in-house laboratories or sent to an outside laboratory (depending on the facilities available and the tests required). Routine profiles usually look at general health, liver and kidney function, and blood cell numbers, but other tests are performed if particular diseases are suspected. Urine tests are often done at the same time.

HORMONE TESTS

Hormone tests are usually performed if a hormonal disease is suspected. Unfortunately, even healthy thyroid, adrenal and sex hormone levels vary widely throughout the day, so single tests are unreliable. Dynamic tests, where levels are measured before and after giving a drug that stimulates the hormone-producing gland, are a better reflection of overall activity. These usually take all day, which requires hospitalisation.

BACTERIAL/FUNGAL CULTURES

Bacterial and fungal cultures are often taken to confirm infection, and to determine which species is involved and which antibiotics or antifungals are effective. Most bacterial cultures take a few days, but fungi and some bacteria can take several weeks.

I tching, scaling and hair loss can develop together or separately, and it is observation of these that normally results in a trip to the local vet.

ITCHING

Itching is usually caused by parasites or allergies. Bacterial and yeast skin infections can also be itchy, but are usually secondary to another skin problem (see Chapter Six).

Dogs commonly indulge in frenzied licking and chewing at a single spot, leaving a hairless, red and moist patch called a hot spot. Allergies, parasites, anal sac problems (see Chapter Seven), painful conditions such as arthritis, and thick or matted coats, particularly in warm weather, are all potential triggers. Treatment involves cleaning and steroid/antibiotic ointments.

Acral lick dermatitis is a condition in which dogs chew at a single spot, usually on the lower leg. Over time, this results in a thickened, darkened, hairless plaque of skin with deep-seated, secondary bacterial infection that requires a long course of antibiotics. Underlying causes include allergies, parasites, arthritis and psychological disorders, which may need referral to a behavioural specialist.

PARASITES

Common parasites include fleas (see Chapter Two), lice, and mites.

- *Sarcoptes:* This causes the highly contagious disease scabies. The microscopic mites burrow in the skin, causing intense irritation and inflammation of the elbows, hocks and ears. Later, there may be wide-spread inflammation, hair loss and crusting.

Mites can be found on skin scrapes, but these are frequently negative, as most dogs harbour very few mites. A blood sample test is now often used instead.

A drug given as drops on the back of the neck is a very effective treatment. All in-contact dogs should be treated. The eggs are resistant to the drug, so treatment should be continued for at least six weeks, to kill newly hatched mites. It is not usually necessary to treat the house, but collars, bedding, etc. should be thoroughly washed. Other treatments include sprays and dips.

- *Otodectes:* This mite is most common in young dogs, causing ear infections with a dark, waxy discharge. It can also affect the head, back and legs.

Otodectes mites are easily diagnosed by otoscope)a device for looking into the ear canal), ear swab or skin scrape. Medicated ear drops (in both ears) and flea drops or sprays are usually successful. Treatment should be continued for four to six weeks to kill freshly emerged mites. All in- contact animals, including cats, should be treated.

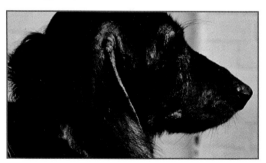

Sarcoptes mites usually attack the face, earflaps, elbows, ventral chest and hocks.

- **'Walking dandruff'** or *Cheyletiella: Cheyletiella* are highly contagious, although many dogs show no ill effects. Affected dogs are usually itchy, with dry, whitish scaling, particularly over the back and flanks.

  Cheyletiella are large mites that can be seen with a hand lens in coat combings as small, moving white specks (hence 'walking dandruff'). They are easily seen on skin scrapes and sticky-tape strips.

  Shampoos are used to remove scale protecting the mites. Long-haired dogs should be clipped to allow proper penetration of the insecticide. All in-contact animals, including cats, should be treated for at least six weeks to kill the newly hatched mites. The house should also be treated, as female *Cheyletiella* can live in the environment for 10 days. Anti-mite shampoos, sprays and drops are available, but some mites are resistant, so you may need to try several products.

- **Lice**: These are uncommon – most infestations are seen in young, ill or kennelled dogs. In large numbers, lice can cause irritation and poor thrift, as well as helping to transmit tapeworms.

  Lice are large, slow-moving insects that are easily spotted. Their eggs ('nits') are firmly glued to the hairs and will catch on a flea comb. Anti-flea and anti-mite products are effective against lice, but treat all in-contact dogs for at least six weeks.

- **'Berry bugs'** or **harvest mites:** These are the larvae of a mite that lives on decaying vegetation, active from July to September. They readily infest dogs (and their owners), causing intense itching.

  The bright orange mites are easily seen between the toes, on the belly, and around the ears. Most anti-flea and anti-mite treatments kill harvest mites, but re-infestation can occur. Long-acting sprays can prevent new infestations, and dogs should be kept away from long grass and woods. Severely affected dogs may need steroids when the larvae are active.

- **Other parasites**: Hookworms occasionally cause itchy, inflamed feet in kennelled dogs. Reactions to other internal worms are very rare. Worm eggs can be detected in faecal samples. Routine worming and faeces removal will prevent problems.

ALLERGIES
Skin allergies are common in dogs, and can range from causing moderate discomfort to severe itchiness. For more information, see Chapter Five.

OTHER CAUSES OF ITCHING
Immune-mediated conditions, infections, internal diseases and certain skin cancers can also cause itching and inflammation. Your vet may suggest tests to eliminate these causes early on.

SCALING
Scaling is a common problem with lots of causes. Dead skin cells are normally shed as microscopic flakes. Scales are large, visible rafts of cells that are not shed properly. They accumulate on the skin and hairs. There are three forms – dry, greasy and mixed, largely determined by the breed. Some breeds (e.g. Cocker Spaniels) have inherently oily skin, while others (e.g. Boxers) have dry skin. Scaling can be a primary problem or it can be secondary to an underlying disease.

SECONDARY SCALING
Secondary scaling is much more common than primary scaling. The underlying cause must be identified. This may be parasites, bacterial and fungal infections, allergies, immune-mediated diseases, some skin cancers,

hormonal or metabolic diseases, follicular dysplasias and low humidity (see below and Chapter Six). Careful examination often reveals clues to the underlying condition, but thorough investigations can be lengthy and costly.

Vitamin, oil and zinc deficiencies are rare with today's variety of off-the-shelf, good-quality diets, but nonetheless, they can still be seen in dogs fed a poor-quality and unbalanced diet. Supplements can help.

English Bull Terriers suffer from an inherited disease called lethal acrodermatitis. Puppies develop inflammation and scaling of the feet and muzzle. Secondary yeast infections are common. Controlling yeast infections and providing a high-quality diet may help, but most dogs do not survive beyond four years.

Fine, silvery-white scaling is characteristic of infection with *Leishmania*, transmitted by sand flies. Rare in the UK, but endemic in southern Europe, it is likely to become more common as more dogs travel. Clinical signs include hair loss, loss of pigment, ulcers and nodules (particularly over the face, nose, ear pinnae and feet), enlarged lymph nodes, fever, and lameness.

Diagnosis is based on antibody tests and identifying the organism in skin and lymph node biopsies. The prognosis is guarded, as many dogs fail to respond to treatment. Dogs travelling to endemic areas should be protected – your vet will suggest a suitable product.

PRIMARY SCALING
Primary scaling is caused by the accelerated turnover and accumulation of skin cells. It is most common in spaniels. Signs first appear in young dogs. The coat becomes dull and they develop focal to generalised scaling. Ear and skin infections are also common.

Diagnosis of primary scaling disorders is difficult,

relying on history, clinical findings, skin biopsies, and eliminating other causes. Many of these diseases are inherited, so affected individuals should not be bred from. There is no cure for primary scaling conditions, but most can be managed with appropriate treatment (see below). Therapy is usually life-long.

- **Vitamin A responsive dermatosis:** This disease is seen in Cocker Spaniels that develop tightly adherent, frond-like scales. Affected dogs are also itchy, malodorous, have patchy hair loss, and bacterial and yeast infections. The disease often responds to vitamin A, but this can have severe side effects and treated dogs should be closely monitored.

- **Sebaceous adenitis:** This is a common problem among Standard Poodles, Vizlas, Akitas, and Samoyeds, and it is occasionally seen in other breeds. Clinical signs include dry skin, tightly adherent, frond-like scales, hair loss, and secondary infections. Several biopsies are usually necessary for diagnosis.

- **Icthyosis:** This is a rare, congenital disorder seen in terriers and a variety of breeds. It can be seen as severe scaling of the skin and footpads, with skin thickening and hair loss from birth. Despite this, more mildly affected dogs can live a relatively normal life with treatment.

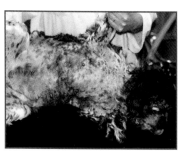

Primary scaling or idiopathic keratinisation defect in a Cocker Spaniel. The accumulated scales have blocked hair follicles and triggered a severe bacterial infection.

LOCALISED SCALING

- **Ear margin scaling**: This is occasionally seen in Dobermanns and other short-coated breeds, with greasy scales on the edges of the earflap. Severe cases may have hair loss and ulceration. Mild cases can be safely ignored, but severe cases require treatment.
- **Naso-digital hyperkeratosis**: This is visible as scaling and crusting of the footpads and nose. It is particularly common in spaniels, but also in older dogs of any breed. Cancers, immune-mediated or metabolic diseases can occasionally cause severe crusting. Treatment is unnecessary unless the nose or pads become cracked and painful.
- **Calluses**: These develop at pressure points overlying the bone, such as the elbows, carpus or wrist, stifle or knee, hock and pelvis. Treatment is not necessary unless they become cracked or infected. Surgical removal is often unsuccessful and not recommended. Homemade elbow/knee pads, and soft beds can help to relieve the dog's discomfort.

MANAGING SCALING

- Feed a high-quality diet. Many dogs benefit from vitamin and essential oil supplements.
- Treat secondary infections promptly. Anti-microbial shampoos can reduce the number of bacteria and yeasts on the skin and help to prevent infections.
- Anti-scaling shampoos that remove excess scales and slow the turnover of skin cells are very effective. Moisturising shampoos are best for dry scaling, whereas de-greasing shampoos are best for greasy scaling. Propylene glycol diluted 1:1 in water is very effective at removing stubborn scales.
- Wet dressings and petroleum jelly are very good on dry, cracked skin. Ointments with salicylic acid

cause thick layers of dead skin to slough away, but these should be used carefully to avoid ulceration.

• Retinoids are very effective in some forms of primary scaling. Although generally well tolerated, side effects include liver and joint problems, dry eyes and dry skin, so treated dogs should be regularly monitored. Retinoids are very toxic to a foetus, and should not be given to breeding animals or be handled by women.

HAIR LOSS

Hair loss (alopecia) is a common problem. However, excessive shedding, albeit annoying, is not significant unless it leaves bare skin. Although there are a wide range of diseases that cause hair loss, the most common cause is self-trauma, so your vet will want to investigate any itching first.

DEMODEX MITES

Often referred to as 'Red mange', *Demodex* are long, thin mites that live in the hair follicles. Puppies acquire them from their mothers. All dogs (and people!) harbour small populations. They can multiply and cause problems in three ways:

• **Localised:** Focal areas of hair loss and scaling are quite common in young dogs, possibly due to puberty. Most will spontaneously resolve.

• **Generalised:** Generalised *Demodex* in young dogs is more serious, with widespread hair loss, scaling, crusting, and secondary bacterial infections.

• **Adult onset:** Adult-onset generalised *Demodex* can be associated with hormonal diseases, metabolic disorders, cancers, steroids or chemotherapy, which suppress the immune system, but most cases are spontaneous, associated with inherited susceptibility.

Affected dogs should not be bred from. Severe cases can be life-threatening.

Demodex mites are usually easily found on skin scrapes or biopsies. Underlying problems and secondary infections should be treated. A dip called amitraz is the mainstay of treatment. Treatment should be repeated weekly until there have been three negative scrapes. This may take several months, and some dogs will require life-long treatment. Systemic drugs (ivermectins) have been used in cases that respond poorly to amitraz, but can be toxic in some dogs.

RINGWORM

Ringworm (or dermatophytosis) is a fungal infection caught from other dogs, cats, and wild animals. Infection is most common among young dogs, causing patchy hair loss, scaling, crusting, and secondary bacterial infections. Older dogs often have underlying immunosuppressive conditions (see above).

Ringworm can be diagnosed by checking for fungi using a microscope or UV light. Fungal culture is also diagnostic, but it may take up to three weeks.

Ringworm in young dogs can spontaneously resolve, but treatment using a combination of antifungal drugs and shampoos is recommended because of the infection risk to humans. Collars, leads, coats, blankets, beds, etc. should be disposed of or thoroughly disinfected with bleach. Dogs are not

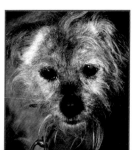

This elderly Border Terrier is suffering from hair loss and scaling caused by dermatophytosis (ringworm). This dog had a hormonal disease that probably allowed the infection to establish.

considered cured until there have been three negative fungal cultures. Stopping too soon is the most common reason for treatment failure.

STRESS

Widespread hair loss can occur some days to weeks following stress, such as pregnancy, nursing, malnutrition, extreme activity, shock, fever, illness, chemotherapy, etc. The skin is essentially quite normal and the coat usually grows back quickly.

CONGENITAL/HEREDITARY/FAMILIAL HAIR LOSS

Congenital diseases are those apparent from birth, but they need not be inherited. Hereditary diseases are those passed on in the genes from one generation to the next. Familial diseases occur in certain breeds or lines, but the genetic basis isn't fully understood. Hereditary and familial diseases are usually, but not always, congenital. Affected dogs and their relatives should not be bred from.

Some breeds, including Mexican Hairless and Chinese Crested Dogs, are 'naturally' hairless. In other breeds, these same genes can cause a major problem!

FOLLICULAR DYSPLASIAS

This group of inherited diseases causes abnormal growth and development of hair follicles. The puppy coat is initially normal, but, over time, it becomes dull, brittle and is lost, predominantly from the trunk. There is often scaling and secondary infection.

The clinical signs and the dog's breed type are highly suggestive of the cause. Skin biopsies will show characteristically abnormal hairs and hair follicles. Unfortunately, there is no specific treatment. Shampoos are used to remove scale and to clear blocked follicles, while any bacterial infections will require antibiotics. Some dogs respond to retinoids (see Scaling, above) and high-quality diets, but the prognosis is generally poor. Affected dogs should not be bred from.

HORMONAL HAIR LOSS
The various hormonal diseases tend to look quite similar. Common features include:
• Symmetrical hair loss
• Dull, dry, faded coat
• Failure to re-grow coat after clipping
• Mild to moderate scaling
• Easily bruised skin and poor wound-healing
• Secondary infections.
   Routine skin biopsies, blood and urine tests can be suggestive, but are rarely diagnostic. Furthermore, no single hormonal test is perfect, and results from several tests are usually combined to confirm a diagnosis. Treatment will vary according to the cause.

Hypothyroidism
Hypothyroidism is caused by a lack of thyroid hormone. Clinical signs are variable, and include hair loss from the collar, nose, tail and trunk, with thickened, pigmented and cool skin. Some dogs have abnormally retained and long hair. Affected dogs are often dull,

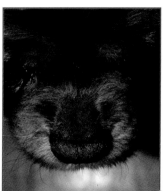

Loss of hair and darkening of the dorsal nose in a hypothyroid Cavalier King Charles Spaniel.

lethargic and overweight, but others are bright and well.

Hypothyroidism is normally treated with thyroid hormone replacement. Prognosis is very good, although life-long treatment and regular monitoring is required.

Hyperadrenocorticism

Hyperadrenocorticism is caused by an excess of steroid hormones – due to a pituitary gland tumour in the brain (which controls the adrenal glands), adrenal gland tumours, or steroid treatment.

Clinical signs include hair loss, excessive drinking and urinating, excessive appetite and weight gain, a potbelly, calcium deposits in the skin (which can be itchy or painful), thin and wrinkled skin, muscle wasting, sugar diabetes, and mood changes.

For dogs on steroids, treatment should involve being gradually weaned off steroids and on to alternative therapies. In naturally occurring cases, drugs are used to limit steroid hormone production from the adrenal glands. Insufficient steroid hormones cause weakness, vomiting and collapse, so dogs are initially hospitalised to establish a safe dose. Steroid tablets can be given in emergencies. The prognosis is reasonable, although pituitary tumours will eventually cause neurological problems.

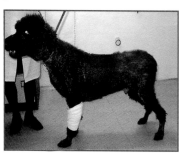

Abnormal coat, hair loss and muscle weakness (note the dished back) in a Standard Poodle with an excess of steroid hormones.

Sex hormone disorders

Sex hormone disorders can result from over- or under-production of the sex hormones. They tend to affect the hind limbs, genitalia, flanks and neck, and can also cause swollen nipples and vulva, signs of oestrus, a pendulous prepuce, swollen anus and tail glands, and black spots around the anus and genitals. Immature genitalia, irregular or absent oestrus and urinary incontinence can be associated with low hormone levels. However, these rarely occur after neutering.

Neutering is curative in cases of over-production due to testicular and ovarian tumours, or functional abnormalities (such as cystic ovaries). Dogs with low levels of sex hormones can be treated with androgens or oestrogens, but this should be closely monitored for any side effects.

MISCELLANEOUS CAUSES OF HAIR LOSS

Alopecia in plush-coated breeds

Plush-coated breeds (e.g. Chow Chows and Keeshonds) can suffer hair loss that starts in adolescence or young adulthood. Initially, the primary hairs are lost, leaving a woolly, puppy-like coat. Eventually, there is complete alopecia and darkening of the skin, although the head and limbs are spared. Diagnosis is based on skin biopsy and eliminating other causes of hair loss. Whether this is a hormonal problem or a follicular dysplasia is not fully understood. Some dogs may have abnormal production of sex hormones from the adrenal glands, and these cases may respond to treatment used in hyperadrenocorticism (see page 27). Other cases can show a good response to either neutering, sex hormones, or melatonin. Spontaneous regrowth and relapse is also seen.

Seasonal hair loss

Seasonal hair loss on the back and flanks is common in dogs. The underlying skin is darker, but otherwise normal. Hair loss and regrowth can vary from year to year. It is possibly linked to changes in day length, although the cause isn't really understood. Some dogs respond to melatonin (the drug used for jet-lag), but no treatment has been consistently beneficial.

Pattern baldness

Pattern baldness is seen in Dachshunds, Boston Terriers and other short-coated breeds. It causes progressive hair loss from the earflaps, head, neck, chest and tail. The skin is usually normal, but the hair loss is permanent.

Alopecia areata

Alopecia areata is a rare immune-mediated condition with irregular areas of hair loss. The skin is otherwise normal. It can be diagnosed on skin biopsies. Spontaneous regrowth is possible, but no treatments have been effective. The cause is not known.

Trauma

Deep wounds or infections, burns, injection reactions (e.g. vaccines, antibiotics and steroids), ribbons, bows and collars can all leave hairless scars.

Clipping

Some dogs fail to regrow hair after clipping. This can be due to an underlying problem, but is most common among Arctic breeds with a very long resting phase in the hair-growth cycle. Vigorous massage and covering the site to keep it warm may encourage early regrowth.

5 Allergies and your dog

Skin allergies are common among dogs, although Boxers, German Shepherd Dogs, West Highland White Terriers and Labradors seem particularly predisposed. There are three main allergic diseases seen in dogs:

• Food allergies/intolerance
• Atopic dermatitis
• Contact allergy.

Food allergy and atopic dermatitis can occur together and are clinically indistinguishable. In a contact allergy, only the skin in contact with whatever is causing the allergy is inflamed. It is important to control parasites and skin infections before investigating possible allergies.

FOOD ALLERGIES/INTOLERANCE

Skin reactions to food are uncommon. It is a misconception that dogs only react to a change of diet – reactions are just as likely after months, or years, on a particular diet. Vomiting and diarrhoea point to food intolerance, but are not always present.

Skin or blood tests can be used, but the only reliable way to diagnose an allergy is by feeding a trial diet for at least six weeks. Consult your vet for advice on this.

If your dog improves on a trial diet, you should offer his normal food. If problems recur, you will then need to feed the trial diet again, adding one new food at a time to identify the cause of the allergy. Commonly implicated foods are beef, dairy products and cereals. Once the foods are excluded, prognosis is excellent.

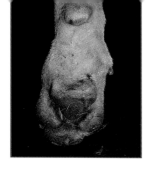

English Bull Terrier with atopic dermatitis. The brown-coloured saliva stains on the feet are caused by excessive licking, resulting in reddening, inflammation and self-trauma of the foot.

ATOPIC DERMATITIS

Dogs with atopic dermatitis react to environmental substances (allergens) that are harmless to normal dogs. Common allergens include house dust mites, danders, insects, pollens or moulds.

Allergens can be identified using skin or blood tests. The prognosis is generally good, but treatment will be life-long. The best results come from combining treatment options, preventing parasite infestations (see Chapter Two), and treating secondary infections promptly (see Chapter Six). Careful observation will allow you to identify and avoid any flare factors, such as irritating substances, central heating, high pollen counts, etc.

ALLERGEN AVOIDANCE

Although it is not necessarily easy, allergens should be avoided where posisble.

House dust mites

- Vacuum and clean regularly. Use fresh bags or a vacuum cleaner with a dust filter.
- After vacuuming, treat all surfaces and furnishings that the dog is in contact with using a proprietary product. (N.B. Read instructions carefully.)
- Keep your pet out of treated rooms for two to three hours, and air rooms thoroughly before allowing the dog back inside.

- Clean the dog's room/bed frequently with a damp mop/cloth. Wash bedding at 60-70 degrees Celsius (140-158 degrees Fahrenheit).
- Keep your dog away from bedrooms, linen stores, washrooms, airing cupboards, stuffed toys or stuffed furnishings. Use mite-proof covers on animal bedding or solid dog beds.
- Carpets harbour mites. Where possible, leave the dog in non-carpeted rooms as much as possible.
- Consider a dehumidifier in modern, insulated homes. These can help to keep the air clear.

Pollens

- Avoid fields, woods, etc., during the hay-fever season.
- Keep weeds out of gardens.
- Keep your lawn short, mowing frequently (but keep dogs away while mowing).
- Don't plant shrubs, etc. near open windows or doors.
- Keep your dogs indoors during high pollen counts, especially early morning and dusk.
- Use an air conditioner.
- Rinse off your dog after he has been outside in or near vegetation.

Moulds

- Avoid, dusty/old foodstuffs, barns, garages, sheds, cellars, straw/hay, compost heaps, lawn cuttings, mats, firewood, wickerwork, etc. (especially if damp).
- Avoid damp rooms (e.g. bathrooms, washing or drying rooms).
- Try not to keep large numbers of houseplants.
- Dehumidifiers and chlorine-based cleaning solutions can help to keep moulds at bay.

IMMUNOTHERAPY

When specific allergens are identified using skin or blood tests, immunotherapy (in which dogs are injected with gradually increasing amounts of allergens) is the treatment of choice. This can take up to 10 months to work and is effective in 60-80 per cent of cases. Initial injections are given at a veterinary surgery, in case of an allergic shock (or anaphylactic) reaction. Fortunately, these are extremely rare.

Immunotherapy is generally well tolerated. Long-term treatment is usually given at home. Most dogs require maintenance injections every one to two months.

IMPROVING SKIN QUALITY

The skin of most atopic dogs tends to dry out, allowing allergens and other irritants to penetrate. Steps to improve skin quality and barrier function include:

- Feeding a high-quality, balanced dog food with adequate levels of essential fatty acids derived from coldwater marine fish (e.g. cod) and plant oils (e.g. evening primrose). Veterinary products are preferred. The initial course is usually eight weeks.

- Regular bathing. Water is very soothing. Moisturising shampoos prolong the effect. Oatmeal shampoos appear to soothe directly, while local application of soothing lotions and creams (e.g. peppermint oil, calamine, menthol and witch hazel), or simply applying ice packs, can help acutely inflamed skin. Sulphur and salicylic acid may also reduce itching, while monosaccharides and piroctone olamine may reduce inflammation and prevent infection. Regular bathing also helps to remove allergens and irritants.

- Regular ear cleaning has a similar effect on the ear canal. It also prevents the build-up of waxy material and inhibits secondary infection.

ANTI-INFLAMMATORY TREATMENTS

Cyclosporin A is highly effective and well tolerated. Transient loss of appetite and vomiting may be seen in the first few days of therapy, but other adverse effects (including persistent vomiting, swelling of the gums, long hair, and wart-like growths) are uncommon and reversible.

A new Chinese herbal therapy compound is very well tolerated and early indications suggest that it is effective in a number of cases. Also, anecdotal reports suggest that gels with aloe vera, tea tree oil, peppermint oil, witch hazel, E45®, Sudacrem®, or ice wraps can be useful for focal inflammation.

Tacrolimus ointment is well tolerated (although not licensed) in dogs. It is messy but useful if lesions are localised to relatively hairless skin, focal lesions, ears and eyes. Topical steroids are far safer than systemic treatment, although they are still absorbed.

ANTIHISTAMINES

Antihistamines are generally safe but can cause drowsiness or stomach upsets. The response depends on the individual, so your vet will try several different drugs to find the best for your dog. Unfortunately, only 25-50 per cent of dogs respond to antihistamines.

ALTERNATIVE THERAPIES

There is great interest in developing other, effective alternatives to steroid treatment in dogs. These include new anti-inflammatory and immunosuppressive drugs, herbal preparations and new forms of immunotherapy. While none can be recommended as yet, it is likely that many more treatments will be available soon. If you are interested in alternative therapies, consult your veterinarian.

Steroids

Steroids are very effective, but they can have major side effects if used for long periods, including hair loss, thinning skin, calcium deposits in the skin, excessive drinking/urinating, excessive appetite and weight gain, liver problems, sugar diabetes and mood changes. Despite this, a low dose given every other day is usually well tolerated and may be necessary if other treatments are not sufficient. Concurrent immunotherapy, antihistamines, essential fatty acids and shampoos can all significantly reduce steroid requirements. Dogs on steroids should have regular checks and long-acting injections should not be used.

CONTACT ALLERGIES

Contact allergic reactions are rare, but can occur in response to dyes, cleaners, eye/ear drops, or shampoos. Irritant reactions can occur with cement, concrete, caustic liquids, cleaners, soaps and shampoos (especially human products).

DIAGNOSIS

Affected dogs need hospitalisation, away from the triggering environment, for up to a week. If the skin improves, suspect allergens are applied to shaven skin for two to three days. The skin becomes inflamed where it has been in contact with an allergen or irritant.

TREATMENT

Ideally, dogs should avoid all further contact with the allergen, which could involve removing carpets, etc. If this isn't possible, steroids, cyclosporin A or other anti-inflammatory drugs may be needed (ointments can be used on non-hairy skin). Immunotherapy is not appropriate for contact allergies.

6 Infections and skin changes

Skin infections are not usually contagious, normally resulting from an overgrowth of bacteria and yeast present on the skin. Such overgrowth often occurs as a result of increased heat and moisture from inflammation and licking, altered sebum, or altered skin cells, etc. Most cases are, therefore, secondary to parasites, allergies, or scaling disorders. They can also be caused by suppression of the immune system, due to puberty, hormonal diseases, cancers, severe illnesses, steroids, and chemotherapy. While these infections will need treating, the bigger challenge is to identify the underlying cause.

BACTERIAL INFECTIONS

Also known as pyoderma or folliculitis, these are frequently very itchy. Infections start with papules and pustules that quickly rupture, leaving patchy hair loss and scaling. In short-haired dogs, lifting of the hairs, making the coat look tufted, is often the first sign. Deeper infections, with draining sinus tracts and ulceration, are seen in more severe cases. These can be quite painful and affected dogs are frequently unwell.

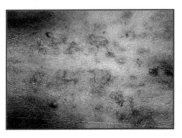

A superficial bacterial infection, with inflammation, spots, pustules, crusts and scale.

YEAST INFECTIONS

Yeasts called *Malassezia* can cause itchy skin and ear infections. Skin affected by *Malassezia* is greasy, hairless, thickened and darkened. Dogs frequently have a musty odour. It mainly affects the muzzle, neck, belly and feet. Basset Hounds are particularly susceptible to *Malassezia* infections.

TREATMENT

Mild infections on the skin surface are usually treated with anti-bacterial and anti-fungal shampoos or washes. Benzoyl peroxide and ethyl lactate are excellent anti-bacterials, and a mixture of chlorhexidine and miconazole is very effective against *Malassezia*. Deeper infections require systemic antibiotics, which are usually given for three weeks, although severe infections may require much longer courses.

Recurrent bacterial infections of unknown cause can be treated with special vaccines prepared from bacterial cultures that stimulate the immune system. Regular anti-bacterial shampoos are also beneficial. Long-term antibiotics are also used, usually at regular intervals (for example – a week on, followed by two weeks off, or every other day, etc.).

CHANGES IN SKIN/COAT APPEARANCE

Most can be safely ignored, but it is always advisable to consult your vet to rule out a more serious cause.

- Permanent or seasonal loss of pigment from the nose is common, but, unlike more serious diseases, it is not associated with loss of the normal 'cobble-stone' appearance of the nose (see Erosions and ulcers, page 41).
- Scars from immune-mediated diseases, infections, injuries, etc. can cause focal loss of pigment.

- Vitiligo is a rare condition associated with the destruction of cells that produce melanin. The skin is otherwise normal, but it needs protection from the sun. It may wax and wane, but there is no treatment. Belgian Shepherd Dogs seem particularly prone to vitiligo.
- A diffuse pattern of dark skin is commonly seen in cases where skin inflammation is due to allergies, skin infections, ringworm and *Demodex,* as well as hormonal diseases.
- Focal patches of dark skin can be caused by benign accumulations of pigment or melanomas. It is important to eliminate malignant melanoma, particularly if the patch is raised or if it appears quite suddenly.

LUMPS AND BUMPS

Lumps and bumps in the skin are caused by either tumours or inflammatory nodules. Tumours are commonly called cancers – although strictly this applies only to malignant tumours. Inflammatory nodules can be infectious or non-infectious (sterile).

The key to diagnosis is deep biopsy of the mass, although cytology can accurately identify some masses. Staining techniques and culture will identify any infectious organisms. Blood and urine tests, ultrasound, X-rays and other tests may also be performed.

Ticks

Ticks are often mistaken for other lumps and bumps. Inflammatory reactions to tick bites are quite common, especially if the body is removed leaving in the head. Ticks should be killed using a flea spray first. They will then either drop off, or they can be gently removed by twisting the head free.

Some of the long-acting flea sprays can protect against re-infestation for up to a month (see Chapter Two). Serious tick-borne diseases are common in continental Europe; any dogs travelling there should be treated regularly to protect them.

Inflammatory nodules

- **Panniculitis**: Sterile or infectious inflammation of subcutaneous fat. Most nodules appear on the trunk. They frequently ulcerate and have a fatty discharge. Most appear spontaneously, but some are associated with drug reactions and immune-mediated diseases. Some respond to vitamin E, but others require steroids or other immunosuppressive drugs.
- **Deep bacterial/fungal infections:** These usually occur following deep wounds or foreign bodies (e.g. grass seeds). Infectious causes can be identified by cytology, biopsy or culture. Many require long courses of antibiotics or anti-fungals and surgery. Foreign bodies must be found and removed.
- **Non-infectious inflammatory nodules:** These can present very similarly to infectious causes, and a careful bacterial and fungal culture is often required. They can be triggered by insect or tick bites and immune-mediated diseases, but are usually spontaneous. Most respond to treatment with steroids, but some require more potent drugs.
- **Juvenile cellulitis:** Common in young puppies, this causes sudden swelling of the muzzle, eyelids, ears and lymph nodes, as well as a thick discharge. Puppies are usually unwell and depressed. It responds very well to steroids and antibiotics, but severe scarring can occur if it is not treated quickly. The cause is unknown, but there is no evidence that it is caused by vaccinations.

Skin tumours

Most skin tumours in dogs are benign. Benign tumours develop slowly, are regular in shape, and are freely mobile. Malignant tumours develop quickly, are irregular, ulcerate, and attach to surrounding tissues. Accurate identification of the tumour is essential to select the best treatment. This may involve combinations of surgery, radiotherapy or chemotherapy.

- **Viral warts:** These are common in young dogs. Most spontaneously regress. Most 'warts' in older animals are actually benign sebaceous tumours, and are only removed if they become inflamed.

- **Histiocytomas:** These are common in young dogs. They are small, red, hairless nodules that rapidly ulcerate, but most spontaneously resolve. They can be removed if they become itchy and inflamed.

- **Histiocytosis:** This is seen mostly in Bernese Mountain Dogs with multiple nodules and ulcers. The course may be rapid with internal involvement, or chronic and fluctuating, but the prognosis is very poor – nearly all dogs will eventually die.

- **Squamous cell carcinomas:** Mainly caused by over-exposure to sunlight, this skin disease manifests itself as thickened, red and scaly patches of skin, which develop into ulcerated and irregular tumours. They are slow to spread, but are malignant and require radical surgery or radiotherapy.

- **Perianal gland tumours:** These are common around the anus and tail in older male dogs. They are usually benign and surgery is curative. They are caused by changes in sex hormone levels, so, without castration, they are likely to recur.

- **Cysts:** Most 'cysts' are benign tumours that have a porridge-like discharge. Most do not need treatment, but squeezing them can cause infection and inflammation – so resist the temptation! Dermoid cysts are congenital, seen in Rhodesian Ridgebacks, Kerry Blues and Boxers. The skin on the back turns inwards. They are surgically removed.

- **Mucinosis:** This can form soft, rubbery nodules, thick skin folds or 'bubbling' of the skin. It is most common in Shar-Peis, where it forms characteristic wrinkles, but can also be caused by hypothyroidism. If necessary, it can be treated with steroids.
- **Urticaria:** Caused by fluid accumulating under the skin. Most are allergic reactions, but spontaneous urticaria is also seen. Steroids or antihistamines will bring down acute reactions.
- **Interdigital cysts:** Red, painful masses that rupture and discharge. Causes include *Demodex* mites, hormonal diseases and foreign bodies, but chronic licking due to allergy is most common. Treatments include antibacterial soaks, flushing and antibiotics. The underlying cause must also be identified.

EROSIONS AND ULCERS
Erosions result from partial, and ulcers from total, loss of the skin. Blisters may be briefly seen before erosions and ulcers develop. The skin can regenerate following erosions, but ulcers heal with scarring. Widespread ulcers can be life-threatening. These lesions often have exudates that dry to form overlying crusts.

Body fold pyodermas
Common in breeds with pendulous lips, facial folds (e.g. Bulldogs) or body folds (e.g. Shar-Peis and obese dogs), and splayed feet (e.g. Bull Terriers). A foul smell is often the most noticeable sign. Antibiotics will clear the infection, but it often recurs. Plastic surgery is the only long-term cure.

Immune-mediated diseases

These occur when the immune system starts to attack the body. Potential triggers include viral and bacterial infections, drug and vaccine reactions, UV light, and cancers, but most are spontaneous. Some breeds appear to be more prone than others. Rough Collies and Shetland Sheepdogs, in particular, suffer from a disease of the skin and muscles called dermatomyositis – affected dogs and relatives should not be bred from.

Mild cases tend to have localised erosions, ulcers and crusting of the nose, face, footpads and scrotum. Initially, the nose becomes paler and loses its normal 'cobblestone' appearance. In more serious diseases, deeper ulcers appear on the nose, face, ears, footpads and the belly. Widespread ulcers with complete loss of skin can be rapidly fatal. Erosions and ulcers can also appear in the mouth, lips, nostrils, eyelids, anus and prepuce or vulva. Affected dogs are often very unwell and secondary infections are common.

Skin biopsies are essential for diagnosis, although specialist techniques may be needed for confirmation. Food trials can diagnose reactions to food additives (although this is very rare). Suspect drugs should be withdrawn. Because of the risks of exposing dogs to suspect drugs to provoke a reaction and confirm the diagnosis, this technique is not recommended.

Treatment of immune-mediated diseases

The goal of treatment is to suppress the immune system enough to put the disease in remission while avoiding side effects. Some drugs are more appropriate for certain diseases than others, so an accurate diagnosis is essential. Unless an inciting cause is found, treatment is often life-long. More potent drugs are used initially to put the disease in remission, and

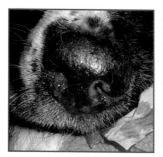

Severe ulceration on the nose of an English Springer Spaniel, caused by an immune-mediated reaction to antibiotics.

less potent drugs with fewer side effects are used to maintain the improvement. Regular check-ups to look for side effects or recurrence of the disease are essential. There are a variety of treatment options.

- **Sunlight avoidance:** See pages 9-10.
- **Steroids:** These are the mainstay of treatment. They act rapidly, and so they are often used at high doses initially. Creams or ointments are useful for local lesions, but tablets are most commonly used.
- **Combination drugs:** Combinations of essential fatty acids and vitamin E, or nicotinamide and tetracycline antibiotics are effective in milder conditions and are relatively free of side effects.
- **High-strength immunosuppressive drugs:** More potent immunosuppressive drugs are used to treat the more serious diseases, and should be used with care. Side effects include liver and kidney problems, bleeding disorders, anaemia and secondary infections. Blood and urine tests should be performed every two weeks during induction and every three to six months thereafter. Despite this, most dogs tolerate these drugs very well.

Prognosis following treatment

With accurate diagnosis, appropriate treatment and monitoring, most conditions carry a good prognosis.

7 Ears, nails and anal sacs

The ear consists of three parts:
- **External ear**: The earflap (pinna) and the ear canal, which form an L-shaped tube leading to the eardrum. It ends at the eardrum, which separates it from the middle ear.
- **Middle ear**: Also known as the tympanic bulla, this bony cavity contains tiny bones that convey sound to the inner ear.
- **Inner ear**: Strictly speaking, this is part of the brain. It controls hearing and balance.

EAR CLEANING

Healthy ears should not need cleaning. However, debris may get trapped in hairy, waxy, or narrow ears, which need regular cleaning. Cleaning is also important in treating and controlling ear infections.
- Always use an ear cleaner recommended by your vet. Not all ear cleaners are appropriate for all ears.

NORMAL HEARING APPARATUS

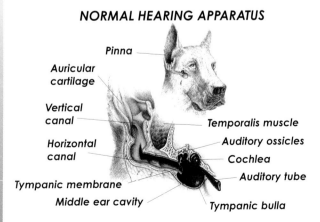

Pinna

Auricular cartilage

Vertical canal

Horizontal canal

Tympanic membrane

Middle ear cavity

Temporalis muscle

Auditory ossicles

Cochlea

Auditory tube

Tympanic bulla

- Follow the manufacturer's instructions carefully. If in doubt, ask your vet to demonstrate.
- Clipping hair from the around the ear can help ventilation and cleaning, but do not pluck hairs or use depilatory creams. Excess hairs can be removed two to three times a year if necessary, with the dog under sedation. Consult your vet.

EAR INFECTIONS

Most dogs develop the odd ear infection from time to time, which quickly respond to treatment with medicated eardrops. However, if your dog develops recurrent ear infections once treatment stops, it is likely that an underlying skin disease is responsible.

- **Foreign bodies:** Common causes of infections, they are usually easy to see and remove at the surgery, but some may require flushing out under sedation.
- **Ear mites:** Common in young dogs (see page 17).
- **Juvenile cellulitis:** Causes a particularly severe otitis externa in young puppies (see page 39).
- **Atopic dermatitis/food intolerance:** The most common causes of recurrent/chronic ear infections in dogs (see Chapter Five).
- **Tumours:** Wax gland tumours are common in older dogs. They can cause infections before the tumour is visible. Most are benign and are surgically excised.
- **Other skin diseases:** Hormonal problems, scaling disorders and immune-mediated diseases can sometimes cause infection.
- **Bacterial/yeast infections:** Rarely initiate ear disease, but can cause secondary infections. They usually respond to medicated eardrops. Infection with *Pseudomonas* bacteria is more serious, with copious greenish, foul-smelling discharge. It frequently requires hospitalisation and specialist treatment.

CHRONIC EAR DISEASE AND SURGERY

Middle-ear infections cause depression, pain, head tilt and difficulty in eating. Ear flushing will remove all the debris from the middle-ear cavity, and long courses of antibiotics may be needed. Surgery is necessary if X-rays show the surrounding bones are involved.

Left untreated or treated inadequately, the ear canals become thickened and narrowed, leading to chronic ear disease with the ear canal eventually becoming blocked. Surgery is then required, although steroids can reverse early changes.

There are two main surgical procedures used when medical treatment has failed or is inappropriate. In a lateral wall resection or vertical canal ablation, either the outer wall or the complete vertical portion of the ear canal is removed, to improve access to the horizontal portion of the ear canal. In a total ear canal ablation, the whole of the ear canal and middle ear cavity is removed. Although more radical, this is necessary in cases of long-standing ear disease. Dogs will be deaf afterwards, and, as with any surgical procedure, there are risks involved. However, generally speaking, the long-term results are very good.

Ear surgery: Vertical canal ablation (left) and total canal ablation (right).

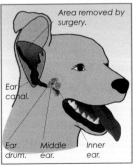
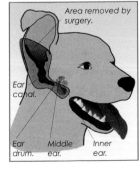

NAIL INFECTIONS

Nail diseases may occur in isolation or as part of a skin condition. Common factors involved include:

- Poor diet or serious metabolic/hormonal illnesses can cause dry, brittle and deformed nails.
- Scars and poor foot conformation can cause deformed nails, which can grow into the pads. Overweight dogs may also have nail problems due to excessive strain on them.
- *Demodex* mites and dermatopytes (ringworm) can cause nail and nail-bed infections, but bacteria and yeasts are usually secondary invaders.
- Immune-mediated diseases can cause discoloration, softening, fracture and sloughing of the nails.
- Some dogs develop soft and brittle nails, or nail loss for no apparent reason.
- Some tumours start in the nail bed. Infection and inflammation may occur before the tumour is seen.
- Caustic or irritant substances can cause nail-bed inflammation and infection.

DIAGNOSIS AND TREATMENT

Amputation and analysis of an affected claw is usually necessary for diagnosis, along with cytology samples.

To treat, all loose and diseased nails should be gently removed and the nail beds kept clean. Treatments useful in spontaneous nail diseases include high-quality diets, mineral and vitamin supplements, nicotinamide and tetracycline antibiotics, and essential fatty acids. Amputation of all the nails has also been successful.

ANAL SACS

The anal sacs are two pouches lying under the skin near the anus. Their malodorous secretion, used for identification and territorial marking, is squeezed out as stools are passed. If the sacs do not empty properly, secretion builds up, dries out, and can become infected.

Common clinical signs include:

- Distended, inflamed and painful anal sacs
- Anal sac abscesses
- Chewing or 'scooting' the rear end along the ground
- Difficulty in passing stools
- Hot spots (see page 16) around the base of the tail.

TREATMENT

Your vet will empty the anal sacs manually, by squeezing them. Antibiotics may also be prescribed if necessary. Severely impacted sacs or abscesses may need flushing.

In some cases, anal sac problems may be recurrent. Long-term prevention can include strict contol of diet (adding fibre if necessary) and weight. Surgical removal is used only as a last resort.

ANAL FURUNCULOSIS

This condition causes extensive, deep ulcers and draining sores around the anus and base of the tail, particularly in German Shepherd Dogs. Mild cases cause few problems, but severe cases are extremely painful. The cause is not understood, but is thought to be related to food intolerance, colitis, and abnormal reactions to bacteria on the skin and rectum.

Your vet will make the diagnosis based on the dog's medical history, clinical signs, and physical examination.

Hypoallergenic diets, steroids and a drug called sulphasalazine will treat any underlying colitis. Cyclosporin A has also been used very successfully. Infected tissues can be surgically excised, although depending on the level of tissue removed, incontinence can result.